SIMPLE PLEASURES

101 IDEAS TO LIVE A RICH LIFE

KRISTI BELLE

INTRODUCTION

The simple pleasures in life can be fleeting if we don't take time to appreciate them—or even create them.

They are the poignant moments that ultimately add up to make up our lives.

Instead of getting caught up in the overwhelm of our modern world, read on to find ways to magically slow down time and increase the pleasure and joy in your life.

It doesn't take winning the lottery or being able to quit your job to make your life 100 percent more pleasurable. You have the power and ability to make your days more satisfying, rewarding and fulfilling.

In this small guide, I aim to make the 101 ideas I share simply jumping off points that will inspire another 100 or so ideas that you can incorporate into your days and life to make your world that much richer in a way that money could never do.

"Simple Pleasures" is an inspirational little book to help you turn the ordinary into extraordinary.

CHAPTER 1

*K*eep a journal.

A wise woman once told me to be careful what I put on paper because written words are powerful.

Of course, after that I became a writer so go figure.

If you are not a natural writer and the thought of scribbling in a notebook every day seems overwhelming then it's time to take another look at what journaling means. Because the reality is that it can mean anything. It can be a way to list your to dos for the day. It can be a place to write poetry. It can be a dumping ground for your most angst-ridden thoughts. It can be a review of your day. It can be a sacred space to hold your darkest emotions and biggest dreams. It can be a place to complain privately knowing that nobody will ever see your concerns.

It can be a place to track your goals or eating habits or spending patterns. It can be a place to write fiction or create a day in the life of a future you in exquisite detail.

You see, for me a journal is all of these things and more.

I put no pressure or expectations on my daily morning journaling. I just make sure I sit down with my Moleskine notebook and write the date and the three things I hope to accomplish on that particular day.

Sometimes a journal page will only contain those things. Other days, I will free-write for four pages about my hopes and dreams, remembering that words on paper are powerful.

Pick out a journal that makes you happy to look at. It could be floral and pink or whimsical with a cartoon character, or simple and black like mine. Grab a pen that makes it a joy to write and set aside five minutes a day to jot your thoughts down.

It might just change your life.

CHAPTER 2

$\mathcal{M}$eal prep and plan.

One of my favorite sayings is Failing to Plan is Planning to Fail.

When it comes to maintaining a healthy diet I've found that this saying counts double.

It's too easy to make poor nutritional choices in a hurry.

To avoid this, every Sunday I meal prep. Because I'm only feeding myself I no longer meal plan, but when I was raising a family, meal planning saved me both time and money by deciding once a week what I would cook for dinner each night and then shopping and meal prepping accordingly. I also made sure to "shop by pantry and refrigerator" first before meal planning so I didn't let any food spoil or go to waste. If something was close to its expiration date, I would make sure to include that in a meal that week. One simple tip that made feeling a family easier was to have Theme Nights. Every Monday was soup or salad. Tuesdays were Mexican food. Fridays were for pizza. And so on.

Nowadays, since I am only feeding myself I meal prep components of meals and then have items prepared I can throw together for a meal during the week. On Sundays, I will prepare proteins for the week which often involves boiling eggs, along with cooking chicken and steak. I might boil rice and use it for fried rice that week. I have cooked batches of quinoa and put that in the refrigerator. I also chop vegetables so it's easy to throw them in a salad or in the skillet for a meal.

Taking the time to meal prep and plan makes it easy to eat healthy.

CHAPTER 3

*C*reate an Inner Italian/Boss Girl/Bestselling Author

This is a perfect exercise for that beautiful new journal you just bought. Ha. But feel free to write this on your computer or tablet.

In this exercise you are going to envision your future or your dream self.

Maybe you love Italian culture so you can write as your Inner Italian Girl. How would she live? How would she dress? Eat? Spend her time?

Or maybe you are a budding entrepreneur. How would your Inner Boss Babe spend her days?

In my case, I began writing a long time ago, long before I became a USA Today bestselling author, how a successful author would spend her days, dress, eat, exercise, and so on.

You are going to write about her in the third person from the minute she opens her eyes until she goes to bed at night. You will detail everything from her habits and routines to her wardrobe and meals. Try to write out her day in excruciating detail. This should be fun. This is the dream life you want to be living. No judgment allowed. This is for your inspiration and your eyes only.

Bonus points if you read this every morning before you start your day.

Here's a prompt to get started. This is also something you could ask yourself every single day as you are faced with the myriad and numerous choices we all have on a daily basis:

What would the hottest and most successful version of you do?

CHAPTER 4

*D*evelop a signature style
If you want to be a memorable woman and also reduce the time and money you spend on your appearance and first impression, take a little time on the front end to develop a signature style.

CHAPTER 5

*I*nvest in your hair.

The first thing we see or recognize about someone. It makes or breaks your look. After spending decades not spending time, money, or energy on my hair, I finally realized (better late than never) how crucial it is to my style and looks. After complaining about how dry and coarse and unruly my hair was, I had a hairdresser tell me a few years ago (during my very far-spaced haircut appointments) that unfortunately this was a side effect of getting older.

She was wrong.

I'd always scoffed at salon shampoos and conditioners and settled for drug store brands, but I decided to invest in high-end products. I not only got the basics, shampoos and conditioners, but also invested in heat protectors and smoothing serums. I also made caring for my hair a priority and know that on the days I wash my hair, that if I blow dry it at a certain point after it has air dried for a while, it will become soft, sleek and manageable until my next wash.

I also make sure to make time for and budget for regularly sched-uled haircuts and color (to dye my gray roots). I no longer wait to call the salon in desperation when I wake up one morning and my hairstyle is no longer working. (How come it happens like that? One day it looks good and then the next morning we realize we needed a haircut a week ago?)

I'm not going to lie - making my hair a priority has elevated my look exponentially.

CHAPTER 6

*C*reate a morning routine

I have an entire book on this.

But in a nutshell: numerous studies have shown that the vast majority of successful people all have similar morning routines.

When I first discovered this, it was as if a secret world had been unveiled. I had no clue that all these people I admired had this one thing in common.

For the most part, they all did most, if not all, of the following things in the morning as their daily routine: exercise, meditate, read, and journal.

So, of course, I had to come up with my own chic take on this.

The interesting thing is that these activities don't have to take a long time.

On those busy mornings, maybe we are doing a quick 10 minute HIIT exercise routine, meditating for 5 minutes, reading for 10 minutes and journaling for 15 minutes. There is no right or wrong.

What matters is carving this time out for yourself before the day - and other people's demands - take over.

The ultimate goal is to set the tone and create the mood for your day. By setting yourself up for a successful day first thing in the morning, you have increased your chances of accomplishing your goals for that day.

CHAPTER 7

*U*se (and learn) Google Calendar. Or a similar planning system

When I first became a self-published author, the amount of time and the number of tasks involved was overwhelming. I not only had to prioritize time to write every day (this is the romantic ideal of being a writer, no?) But I had to figure out time to do all the other myriad business tasks of being self-published.

The list was never ending. I had to arrange editors, proofreaders, an advanced reading team, social media posts, paid promotions, cover designers, copy for the back of the book, the actual formatting and uploading to the publishing platforms and on and on and on.

Without a printed planner or Google Calendar system, I would not have been able to do it.

For a few years I loved the idea of a printed planner and became a planner junkie, outlining what I would do for chunks of each day.

Eventually I moved to scheduling my life on a Google Calendar. I love the electronic version and use it to organize not only my writing life, but my personal life as well. For instance, I can use it for recurring appointments. I know that every Friday is Finance Friday where I sit down and go over my finances. Saturdays and Sundays are for household tasks that appear repeatedly on my calendar each weekend such as watering the plants, refilling the dog food canister, meal prep and other chores.

My life is run by an electronic calendar and I have never felt more organized and never been as successful as I am now.

The proof is in the pudding.

CHAPTER 8

*E*levate your lingerie game.

When I turned 50 I went to the most luxurious lingerie store in the state of Minnesota and walked out with $1,000 worth of the most exquisite, to-die-for matching bras and underwear sets. Three to be exact. Worth every penny.

Hey, you don't turn 50 every day.

But on a regular basis, I invest in the most comfortable lingerie for my lifestyle and body. Recently that has been Victoria's Secret bras because I found an underwire style that doesn't leave bruises on my ribs like some. (Don't ask. I have no clue why they do this to me.) For the past decade, my staple underwear has been the Hanky Panky original rise lace thongs. I've tried to deviate and buy similar ones but there has never been one other brand that has even come close to the quality and comfort of these underwear. So I'm a die-hard fan for life.

I baby all my lingerie by washing them in a lingerie bag on hand wash and then hanging to dry.

I am a strong believer that elevating your lingerie, even if you are the only one who ever sees it, is a game changer in your confidence level.

CHAPTER 9

*L*earn to meditate.

As I mentioned in the section on morning routine, the majority of successful people in the world do some form of meditation. I attempt to do it every day. I say attempt because I sometimes skip a day. And to be honest, on the days I do sit down to meditate, I don't often make it until my 10 minute timer goes off. But they call it a meditation practice for a reason. Some are better than none. And the benefits of meditation are proven. (I could write a whole book on this, but I'm sure you can delve deeper if you are interested.)

Needless to say, one thing I adore about the benefits of meditation is there is no black-and-white right-or-wrong method. There are so many different ways to meditate.

You can hop on YouTube and do a guided meditation. You can sit quietly for ten minutes and let your thoughts run rampant. You can simply focus on your breath. You can chant a mantra.

For me, I began by using Headspace. This app has a free and paid version. The first year I paid so I can learn ways to meditate for different situations.

Now, I most often sit down and try to focus on my breathing for ten minutes. Occasionally I might find some calming music or an inspirational guided meditation, but on a daily basis, I usually am just quieting my thoughts.

This alone is huge.

Doing this is free, can be done anywhere, and has incredible benefits.

CHAPTER 10

*W*alk at least 20 minutes a day.

There is a trend on TikTok right now saying if you want to be in amazing shape all you have to do is get on a treadmill, set the elevation to 12, the speed to 3, and walk for 30 minutes every day for a month.

I'm not sure if this is true or not, but I do believe in the crazy benefits of walking for 20 minutes every day.

I subscribe to a theory that I first heard from Tim Ferris. It's called the MED and stands for Minimum Effective Dose.

The idea is to use your time and energy on the minimum activity that will bring you the maximum results.

Walking for 20 minutes every day is the perfect example of this. Studies show this is the minimum exercise you need to gain the maximum health benefits.

Sign me up.

If you can't walk outside (and you don't have a damp, dark basement with a crappy old treadmill like me - ha) you can walk in circles in your living space for 20 minutes. Not ideal but doable. Sometimes, in between writing sprints I will fast walk around my small house to get my walking in.

Walking is free. It's a mood booster. It's good for your head, heart, and health.

CHAPTER 11

*U*se sunscreen religiously.

If for no other reason, use sunscreen every day to avoid the possibility of having huge chunks of your flesh taken off your face when you grow older. And that's the cancer that usually doesn't kill you. The other one, also caused by sun exposure, could. And it's one of the most deadly cancers if not caught early.

Melanoma runs in my family and it's no joke.

Okay. But all seriousness aside, my daughters ask me how come I look so much younger than most other women my age - 54 - and I truly believe there are two major factors. And only one that I - and everyone else - can control. The first is genetics. The second is my religious use of sunscreen since I was a teenager.

Hey, I like bronze skin as much as the rest of us, but that's what fake tanning lotion is for in my opinion.

I live in Minneapolis, Minnesota where winter seems to last for 8 months of the year. And I use sunscreen 365 days a year. It's the first thing I put on when I sit down to do my makeup. I now put it on my neck and decollete and am kicking myself for not doing this earlier as my chest has sun damage. I also regret not using it on the back of my hands, which have damage, as well, with unsightly age spots. They look old. But luckily my face looks much younger than they do since I've always prioritized facial sunscreen.

Find a brand that feels great on your skin and make it part of your daily routine.

CHAPTER 12

*C*reate a marketing list. You can have one list with pantry items you should always have stocked. Another list for items you pick up weekly. A list for monthly. And so on.

I am obsessed with developing systems and processes to make my life run smoother, to free up time for the things I love and to save money.

Having a marketing list does all those things.

At one point, I had a printable list that had my pantry, freezer, and refrigerator staples listed. I had it hanging on the refrigerator and each time I ran out of something, say, butter, I would circle it on the list. Then before I went shopping, I would review my pantry, freezer, and refrigerator to see what staples were missing and circle those.

Sitting down with my list I would meal plan and then add items I needed to buy at the store for that week's menu.

Armed with this list I would go to the market. I rarely bought anything that wasn't on the list, so my visit was efficient and less costly than if I had just gone willy nilly and started throwing items in my shopping cart.

If you are a coupon shopper, you could sit down with the weekly circulars from the markets and use sale items to meal plan, as well.

Nowadays, I have a pretty standard way of eating each week and so I have 99 % of those items set up as "repeat" items in my Amazon-Fresh shopping cart. Once a week, my Google Calendar reminds me it is shopping day and so I go in and fill out that shopping cart and have my groceries delivered. I never go over budget as I can see exactly what the food items cost. If I have, say, extra eggs left over, I may not buy those that week and might use the budgeted money for another item.

This method saves me time, money and energy and allows me to focus on healthy eating.

CHAPTER 13

*D*evelop a budget.

As mentioned above, I adore sticking to a budget.

I've done many methods of budget keeping over the years including using a small notebook I carry around to track expenses, a fancy app or even an accounting book.

Nowadays I've created my own spreadsheet online that allows me to track all my expenditures and bills. I have a system set up that also shows me my net worth on a daily basis.

Every day I record my expenses from the day before and check in on my financial goals, debt, and savings.

My system allows some flexibility. For example, I can take some money out of my restaurant budget if I want to buy an unplanned clothing item.

By having a realistic amount of money budgeted for various items, I don't have to feel guilty about getting manicures, pedicures, monthly haircuts, or a new pair of high heels.

As a side note, I also keep a list of items to buy and rarely deviate. It takes something pretty important to buy something not on my list.

I have budgeted and planned for these expenses and made adjustments to make them happen.

It's all about priorities.

Sticking your head in the sand if you are in debt is not going to help and will very likely make it worse as debt might continue to build.

Staying on track of your finances is chic and the way to build wealth.

$\mathcal{M}$ ake goals.

Goals are a road map telling your brain where to go.

Writing down your goals also helps you to keep track of your progress - or reveals when you are going off track. Basically they help keep you focused.

You can't make any progress if you don't know where you want to go.

I know there are so many different ways to write your goals. Some people recommend you write them in the form of an affirmation. Some people say write your goals as if they have already happened, such as writing an "end of the year" letter to yourself talking about how great it was to achieve all your goals. Some people say write your goals down and read them every day. Others say write down your goals and set it aside until the end of the year.

Others want you to track goals with a daily habit tracker. Others say you have to have daily, weekly, monthly, biannual, annual, five-year, and ten-year goals. Or that you can just make a vision board at the beginning of the year and that does the trick.

I'm a firm believer that it doesn't matter how you write your goals - just that you have them - and have them written down somewhere to review periodically.

CHAPTER 15

$\mathcal{W}$rite out your perfect day. Then take steps to make it real.

This is a bit like making goals but leans more toward visioning your perfect life. A bit like what would the hottest and most successful version of me do, but laid out by activities and tasks.

For instance, instead of writing about my Inner Italian Girl, instead I'm writing what the Kristi of today does on an ideal day.

My day begins with my morning routine, leads right into making an espresso and sitting down to write for four hours. Then I have lunch, go for a walk, and then do entrepreneurial business tasks for the next four hours. I then eat an early dinner and spend the rest of my day with family and friends.

This didn't happen overnight. I've been a full-time author for 9 years. My days weren't always this ideal. There were years when I had to still do business until I fell asleep. But with the time and energy put into my career, I've worked hard to design my life and live my perfect day every day.

What is your perfect day? Think about it. Right it down and then look at what would need to happen to make it your reality like I have.

CHAPTER 16

*C*reate an evening routine.

      I'm a firm believer that sleep is essential for optimal success and health.

I have an evening routine that helps me prepare for the next day and wake up energized and ready to go.

I often sit down with my journal and review my day.

I also am vigilant about turning off electronics in all forms at least an hour before my set bedtime. Blue light is a thing! We need to honor our circadian rhythms.

I also keep a set bedtime and wake time.

Last night I went to a concert and was home two hours past my bedtime so there are exceptions to this, but I make them rate. Because I believe that sleep is so critical I am tempted to try to sleep in to make up for lost time, but I also believe I should keep a standard wake up time every single day so my solution is to have a short nap the next day.

My phone lets me know when it is "wind down" time for bed and then turns off all notifications during my sleep hours.

In the morning, my phone greets me with a Good Morning message and the temperature for the day when I awaken.

I also make sure my room is pitch black. I am trying to maximize my ability to sleep as much as possible. This involves cutting off the copious amount of water I drink every day a few hours before bed time so I don't wake in the night to use the restroom.

Part of my evening routine is that no matter how tired I am I will never go to bed without removing my makeup and applying tretinoin cream to my face.

Once you establish an evening routine, it becomes a habit and you won't have to think twice about it.

CHAPTER 17

*F*ocus on eating 7-10 cups of vegetables a day.

Do you struggle with eating healthily? Do you want to lose weight? Do you want to gain weight? Do you fight an addiction to sugar and processed food?

Do you follow a strictly KETO or vegan or gluten-free diet?

None of this matters for what I'm recommending.

The number one best thing you can focus on is to eat as many vegetables as you can in a day. Ideally, you will have a variety of vegetables in different colors with leafy greens as your mainstay each day and then other vegetables added in for variety.

This helps your body so much. Not only are you filling it with nutrients, if you strive for 7 to 10 cups a day, you also are filling yourself up on healthy food that is satisfying. This will help reduce cravings for other foods and frankly, give you less room for the unhealthy foods.

If you do nothing else, this will increase your health tenfold.

CHAPTER 18

*P*erfect your skin-care regimen.

As I mentioned early, start your skin-care regimen each day with sunscreen. And then decide what works and what doesn't to make your skin glow.

Some people swear by Vitamin C serum. Others use a lotion with Retin-A.

Some people moisturize religiously. I can't or my face will break out.

I know many women who have elaborate routines involving a cleanser, a toner, and an astringent after.

For me, I have discovered, after decades of overspending on skin care, that for me, simple is better.

At night, I soak a cotton pad with eye makeup remover and gently pat my eye makeup with it until it comes off. Then I wash off my makeup with a little warm water and dove soap. Then I rinse.

Then when I get into bed, I use some tretinoin cream, which is prescription level and basically a generic form of Retin-A.

While I drink my coffee, I apply caffeine-infused eye masks under my eyes. Then before my shower, I use oil and my gua sha. (More on that later.)

In the morning, I blot my face with a warm washcloth but don't use any soap or cleanser. I then begin my makeup routine, beginning with sunscreen, of course.

CHAPTER 19

*B*uy less but buy the best.

This is pretty self-explanatory but worth mentioning.

It's always better to save for the quality item if you intend to get a lot of use out of it.

For instance, let's look at clothing purchases.

If you are buying a tee-shirt in a trendy color that you know you may not wear the following summer, it makes sense to buy something cheaper and more affordable.

However, if your uniform involves you wearing the same style of form fitting white tee-shirt every day under your blazer at work, then it would be worth investing in a higher-quality tee-shirt.

Say you are looking to replace your vehicle. You have $20,000 to spend. In this case, maybe at first you think buying best would be an old Range Rover with tons of miles on it. But after carefully considering the repair costs of an older vehicle of that sort, your best might be using that same money to buy a quality vehicle that will not cost you money in the long run.

So what is best can be arbitrary and really boils down to what is best for you and your budget and lifestyle.

CHAPTER 20

Get off sugar and processed foods.

Sugar is addictive to me. Maybe you might disagree but the more sugar I have the more I want. It doesn't do anything to benefit my health. And its benefits are crazy short-lived. I enjoy it for the few seconds I'm eating it and sometimes that's enough. But unless it's an amazingly delicious treat, I often regret it immediately afterward as my blood sugar spikes, my heart races and my skin later breaks out.

Not worth it.

Processed foods make me feel sluggish and gross after I eat them and are never fulfilling.

I think sugar and processed foods can be had but in very limited quantities.

This is of course my opinion, but I think they only hurt us.

If food doesn't taste delicious AND makes me feel good and energetic afterwards, it's not worth it for me.

CHAPTER 21

*L*earn techniques to de-stress. Have a toolbox of things to do to help you eliminate stress out of your life. Have long-term solutions but also in the moment ways to destress.

Stress is not only aging, but it's dangerous to your health. Chronic stress is linked to all sorts of ailments.

Anything that can be done to alleviate stress is golden.

My short-term fixes involve going for a walk, listening to music I love, taking a long drive, meditating, taking a nap, journaling, writing out my problems on paper, watching a movie that makes me laugh, calling a friend … the list goes on and on.

Take some time to make your list of toolbox items to turn to when you are anxious or stressed.

In addition, long-term solutions are needed.

Maybe it's therapy. Maybe it's lifestyle changes, such as giving up alcohol, changing jobs, and so on.

While some techniques are universal, many of these are specific to you and your situation, lifestyle and personality.

CHAPTER 22

Study yourself and learn your body type and what style flatters it.

Do you know what your body type is?

I'm slightly pear-shaped where I hold my weight a little bit more in my hips. My waist is smaller and my breasts are too.

I know that a dress without a waist makes me look like a blob.

In addition, I know that a dress with a gathered waist makes my backside look enormous.

At the same time, I know that a dress that is tight on the bodice, nips at the waist and slightly flares as it drops to my knees is most flattering.

However, my friends have a different body shape and those shapeless, waistless sheath dresses that fall above her knee make her look like a statuesque goddess.

Set up your camera with a timer and take pictures, front and back, of all your outfits. Analyze them and figure out what styles best flatter your body type.

This will save you money, time and energy down the road when you go shopping and also help build your confidence as you learn to only dress in clothes that flatter you.

CHAPTER 23

*D*on't complain.

It only makes you look bad.

I'm not talking about sticking up for yourself or someone else when there is an injustice or something that is unfair or wrong.

I'm talking about just complaining about things you (and often nobody) can control.

For instance, I learned a long time ago that it only made me look back to complain about Minnesota's bitter cold winters.

Nobody cares. I obviously choose to live here so bitching about it only makes me look bad.

And it doesn't change a darn thing.

If you are just bursting with outrage, pull out that journal you bought in the beginning of this book and write every single little thing that drives you crazy and then close the covers of that book and let it go. It only bothers you. It creates stress that nobody needs.

If you absolutely must complain to someone else, do it behind closed doors, privately to someone you trust to keep it mum.

CHAPTER 24

*B*ase the foundations of your wardrobe on neutrals.

Here is a simple trick to save time, energy and money. (Have you figured out that the last sentence is my motto in living artfully - everything I do is geared to save time, energy, and money.

By using neutrals to build the basics of your armoire you will be able to coordinate all of your clothing easier. Your existing clothes will do double time. Neutrals also are timeless and can be worn more frequently. If you have a pink leather motorcycle jacket, people will notice if you wear it all the time. However, if you have a black blazer and wear it several times a week nobody will even notice.

Along with using neutrals for the basics, it also helps to keep all your other clothing in a predetermined color palette that will match with the neutral colors you've picked.

For instance, you might now want to buy royal purple tops if your foundation items are warmer neutrals such as beiges. However, if your neutrals are blacks or navies, the cooler purple color might look striking instead of odd.

Also, making neutral colors the foundation of your wardrobe will also save you money on buying shoes as you can make your shoes neutrals as well.

CHAPTER 25

*D*ress up daily. Even when you are working remotely at home, take time to dress each day.

Even if your version of getting dressed is your fanciest leggings and a nice t-shirt. It still creates a sense of self worth. The problem is when you pull on your rattiest clothes because you are working at home. Or worse, stay in your pajamas. Every day. Of course once in a while won't hurt, but I still think it affects your attitude and gives your subconscious the wrong impression.

When I get dressed up and put on makeup to sit alone at my dining room table and write each day, I am programming my brain to sit down and work the same as if I left the home and worked in an office.

Not to mention if I have to run out of the house for any reason, I'm ready to go at any point.

CHAPTER 26

*M*ake your home a safe haven.

If you need to, create rules that detail the expectations you have for people inside your home.

This might be a list just for you. Or if you have kids, you can share it with them.

For instance, we don't call names in this house. We take off our shoes when we enter during the winter. We picked up after ourselves, leaving a room as we found it. We chip in to keep the household running smoothly.

In addition, declutter your home of items you don't need or use.

In my case, doing this also clears my head.

My home is full of the things that make me happy.

When I walk into my place I am filled with a sense of calm and peace.

I make sure my home has soft, ambient lighting, lots of leafy plants, fresh flowers, cozy and soft fabrics such as velvets and faux furs, books, candles and fairy lights. All things I love!

CHAPTER 27

*L*earn how to incorporate Hygge into your life. The Danish are one of the happiest people in the world.

This is a little bit of a tangent from the above item, but this philosophy involves embracing the coziness of the colder and darker months.

It involves tactile fabrics, such as warm fuzzy socks, lots of candles, hearty soups and stews and friends over for good conversation.

Pick up a book on Hygge (pronounced Hoo-gah) or search for some articles and find ways you can incorporate this sense of coziness into your life.

It's about slowing down to appreciate the small pleasures in life with those you love.

Even if it's your furry children. You can spend quality time and enjoy life in your cozy home no matter what is going on outside.

CHAPTER 28

*D*eclutter on a regular basis. It could be weekly, or even seasonally.

Go through each room in your house and pick out a few things that you don't use or love and set them aside in a box for a month. If they aren't items you use seasonally and you don't miss them, you can donate or sell after a month or two out of your sight.

Do this on a periodic basis to keep your home clutter free.

You can do this with the items in your closet and too. You can also use it for your makeup and skin care products. Every single area of your life can be decluttered.

It will make you feel more free and clear headed.

CHAPTER 29

*D*on't play small.

Particularly if you are a woman, remember to not play small.

Take up space.

Be your wild and wonderful self.

You don't need to dumb yourself down or dampen your light for anyone or any reason.

Speak out.

Be passionate.

Love deeply.

Laugh with all your being.

Life is short. Life it to the fullest.

CHAPTER 30

$\mathcal{A}$dd plants into your environment.

Plants are a way to add a beautiful touch to your environment. They add a pop of nature to your indoor space and infuse the air with much needed fresh oxygen, as well.

They can be big or small, but this addition of greenery brings life to any home.

CHAPTER 31

*N*ever apologize inappropriately.

We women especially find ourselves doing this.

It's ingrained in our culture to say sorry for the dumbest reasons. Sorry, but it's true.

We say sorry when we accidentally brush somebody in public. We say sorry if we are about to offer a different opinion than ourselves. We say sorry for no good reason.

I was once in line at the post office when the clerk asked the woman if she had anything else to mail and the woman said, "I'm sorry, I have another box."

What? Why was she sorry? Why did she feel the need to say that?

Later that day at the nail salon, the clerk asked the woman if she had trimmed her

Learn to only say sorry when you have done something wrong.

CHAPTER 32

*C*onsider extending your wardrobe palette into your home.

Just for fun, consider taking your colors you use in your wardrobe and incorporate them into your home. For instance, my wardrobe palette consists of blacks and charcoal gray and navy with an occasional pop of turquoise or emerald or amethyst. During the summer almost all of my shoes have leopard print in some way.

My jewelry is all silver except for a special lucky piece.

For my home, I have a large black wood dining room table with navy velvet chairs. My leather couch and chair are dark brown (so not exact) but I have leopard print faux fur throw pillows.

My chaise lounge and other faux fur blankets and pillows are charcoal gray.

The vast majority of my picture frames are silver or pewter. Same for my candlestick holders and candelabras.

My many plants are in either black or white pots and my bedding is all white with charcoal gray faux fur throws (see not exact since I don't wear white).

So you get the idea. Everything in my home is my style to a tee.

CHAPTER 33

*E*mbrace the natural patina of vintage and used items. The soft worn leather couch. Tarnished candelabras. The well-loved vintage set of carnival glass goblets.

Adding small touches of vintage and used items adds a unique old world money element into your style.

I would much rather have a vintage Chanel bag than a brand new shiny one. And although I love my new navy faux fur coat, the vintage brown one from 1970 is even more chic and commented on by other women.

An antique desk or chair or piano adds a unique stylish touch to your home. What about a stack of old hardcover books? One of my favorite decor items (because it's cool but also because I'm a writer) is a black 1940 Royal typewriter that actually works and sits on a buffet side table.

Vintage and used items add a personal touch to your home and elevate it from basic to stylish.

CHAPTER 34

*D*evelop an efficient method and systems and processes to deal with paperwork that comes into your home and inbox.

I have an office type inbox where I pile bills and paperwork that need to be dealt with. Once a week I designate a day to go over that inbox.

Most of my bills are electronic and set up on automatic withdrawals, which has saved me more time than anything else in this area.

I also have an email inbox system that helps me categorize and organize my emails so I never have more than 10 unanswered emails at a time.

My emails are filed into category inboxes: "Coming Up" and "To do" and "Kids" are just a few examples.

My work email has a vacation responder set up that says because I am busy writing books I only check that email address on Fridays. Then I set aside time on Fridays to go through all the reader emails.

CHAPTER 35

*U*se cord organizers. to clean up the mess of cords behind.
I learned this at today years old. I can't believe what a difference this makes in the way the rooms in my house look. Such a simple, easy fix.

Find the cord collectors that suit your needs best and get them already!

CHAPTER 36

*O*nly buy from a list.

  This saves costly mistakes and buyer's remorse.

If I want something badly and it's not on my list yet, then I force myself to write it on my list and wait 24 hours. If I still want it badly after that time, and I have the money for it, then I can buy it.

This method keeps me out of debt and helps me stick to a budget.

In addition, it prevents impulse buys that are a waste of money and full of regret.

CHAPTER 37

*R*ead 10-15 minutes a day. Inspiration and motivational books or articles are my preferred reading material.

I incorporate this reading into my morning routine.

But I also love reading fiction so I enjoy making reading fiction part of my bedtime wind down routine when I am avoiding any electronics for the hour before bed.

Reading is a great way to educate yourself and escape for very little money - especially if you have a library card.

CHAPTER 38

$\mathcal{U}$se caffeine-infused eye masks under eyes. Can apply while you drink your morning coffee if you drink coffee.

As you saw, this is something I mentioned in my skin-care routine.

It's a simple, chic little habit that feels luxurious and helps prevent and treat any dark circles and bags. I love the habit of wearing them during my morning coffee.

I recently was traveling and had a layover in the Nashville airport. I decided to make use of my time there and stopped in at a nail salon for a pedicure I had planned a few days after my trip.

While I was getting my pedicure in the massage chair I also asked for some eye masks.

So luxurious. And a great way to look fresh after a day of traveling.

CHAPTER 39

eep a gratitude list.
Some people say that the secret to happiness in life is gratitude.

Over the years, I've incorporated keeping a gratitude list into my journaling during my morning routine. It has taken shape in many forms. It has been a list of everything I could think of at one time. It has been formed with affirmation words. But most recently I've discovered my most favorite method yet.

Each day I list three things I am grateful for that happened in the last 24 hours. This makes me think and appreciate the small things even more.

Because before I heard about this method I would often say the same exact things day after day. And while that isn't necessarily bad, this has made me even more appreciative of the small things in life.

CHAPTER 40

*D*rink water. Mostly.

Once upon a time I lived on water, coffee, and wine.

Then I realized that wine hates me. Not really. I discovered that my body hates wine. It treats alcohol like poison now that I'm in my 50s. And that's okay by me.

So now I live on water and coffee.

And very rarely, sparkling water.

I find there is no need to drink anything else. I'm certainly not going to have drinks with tons of chemicals, calories and dyes.

I see no reason for that.

And I believe that my skin is soft and supple year round because I prioritize my water intake every day.

CHAPTER 41

*D*evelop a chore list.

To keep my household running smoothly, I use my google calendar to keep track of my chores.

For instance, on Fridays and Tuesdays, I do my personal laundry. On Saturdays, I wash household items, such as towels and sheets.

On Saturdays, I sweep and dust and clean the bathrooms.

On Sundays, I meal prep.

On Thursdays I grocery shop. Ahem, on Amazon, as I mentioned.

I have days on the calendar where I do monthly chores such as wipe down all the baseboards or clean all the pictures in the frames.

Keeping track of all this electronically makes it painless and easy to keep a clean, organized home.

CHAPTER 42

*T*ake your supplements.

The vitamins you take are very personal so I suggest you check with a nutritionist or doctor for what you need in particular.

I can say that I take the following supplements daily as a 54-year-old woman: fish oil, vitamin D, a multi-vitamin, calcium, magnesium, zinc, N.A.C, CoZ10, and a probiotic.

I make sure I research the brands I buy extensively.

I truly believe that my immune system is stronger than it's ever been because of the supplements I've determined work best for me.

CHAPTER 43

*C*hoose your MIP each day.

When you take out your pretty little journal each day for your morning routine, put a list of the Most Important Projects you will do that day.

Ninety-nine percent of the time my first MIP is Write 3,000 words. Then I go from there. I keep my MIP limited to three items.

If I do nothing else that day except those three items then I consider the day a win.

Having these MIP helps keep me focused and helps me prioritize the things that need to be done to move the needle.

CHAPTER 44

*P*rioritize manicures and pedicures.

It took me a long time to realize that investing in having nice nails is worth it.

I am awful at home manicures and pedicures but hated spending a small fortune at the nail salon.

But as a woman in my 50s I decided that one thing I will no longer do is a home manicure.

I will save and budget to have my nails done at a salon. They look gorgeous and polished and professional and make me happy every time I see them.

WHen someone sees my nails I do not cringe in embarrassment. I know that taking care of my nails shows I take care of myself in other ways, as well.

CHAPTER 45

*B*uy investment pieces for your curated wardrobe.
Think about what pieces in your wardrobe are timeless and curate investment pieces over the years. Save and buy the best.

For instance, instead of going through several small crossbody bags for the next decade, I am saving to buy the Saint Laurent Kate bag that will last me for the rest of my life if I so choose.

I also decided that instead of going through several different blazers each year - a staple of my wardrobe - that I would save up and invest in the ultimate blazer - a Veronica Beard blazer. I will wear this unparalleled beauty for a lifetime.

I also invested in a Dolce & Gabbana form fitting sheath and a black Diane Von Furstenberg wrap dress. These items will never go out of style and are worth spending a bit more on as I know I will keep them for years.

CHAPTER 46

*L*og off from work each day. This is especially important if you work at home or are self-employed.

The need to do this became clear during the pandemic when lines between work and home life became fuzzy.

To avoid burnout and to maintain your quality of life consider creating a ritual where you sign off or log off from your work day. Imbue this moment with a ritual such as logging off your laptop, putting it away and then making yourself a cup of tea. Something that can signal the shift from work to home life.

This small habit can bring more pleasure into your life in a simple way.

CHAPTER 47

$\mathcal{D}$ecide on and wear a uniform.

One of the best decisions I ever made regarding my style was to pick a uniform and stick to it. This has saved me - you know what I'm going to say - time, energy and money.

I am confident that I always look good and am always dressed appropriately for the activities in my life.

My uniform has changed over the years.

One summer I only wore sleeveless, knee-length sundresses.

Another summer, I lived in black capri pants and navy scoop neck tees.

This summer I lived in black maxi dresses.

During the past two winters my uniform has been slim black jeans, boots, and Uniqlo scoop neck tees in black with either a blazer or cashmere sweater over them.

I love my uniform and it makes getting dressed every day automatic and easy.

CHAPTER 48

$\mathcal{U}$se lighting in your home to create ambiance.

I'm a big fan of creating a mood through light.

I never turn on bright lights in the morning until I'm through with my morning routine.

Instead, I use fairy lights, LED lights and candlelight to navigate my morning activities.

In the dark days of winter, my home is always cheery and glowing with these lights as soon as the sun sets.

Harsh lights ruin the vibe in my home and I would rather have no lights at all.

Consider creating your own welcome ambiance through your home lighting.

CHAPTER 49

*P*ersonalize your art.

I'm a big believer in using photos as art.

When each of my daughters had their senior pictures taken, I had the best photo blown up and made into a large canvas print. They hang side by side and make me smile every time I see them.

I have two pieces of art in my home that were given to me by artist friends. They mean the world to me. Three of my favorite art pieces are prints I had custom framed. They are gorgeous colorful reproductions of original posters celebrating festivals in Spain that my mother brought home for me after visiting that country. And the upstairs hallway in my house has my favorite artworks - they are framed artwork that my daughters did growing up.

In addition, I have autographed author photos from two of my favorite authors that are framed and hung in places where I will be inspired.

There is not one single piece of art in my home that is not meaningful.

I would never in a million years go into a store and buy a piece of art to match my home.

Each piece, carefully collected over the years has meaning and significance.

They fill my heart with joy every time I see them.

Isn't that what art is supposed to do?

CHAPTER 50

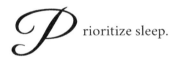 rioritize sleep.

CHAPTER 51

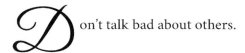 on't talk bad about others.

CHAPTER 52

Use big words around children (and others).

CHAPTER 53

*E*stablish rituals. Daily ones. Weekly ones. Monthly. Seasonally. Annually.

Pinterest Saturday mornings. Annual visit to the apple orchard.

CHAPTER 54

Take up space.

CHAPTER 55

*D*ecorate with meaningful objects.

This is a bit like personalizing your art, but applies to all your decor. When I feel like redecorating the first thing I do is look at useful objects or meaningful objects I already have in my home. For instance, I love books so a stack of black or white books makes a base for an arrangement. I might put candles on top of them or something else meaningful such as a few of the oversized chess pieces from a set I played with as a child.

I don't buy or set out anything for decor that doesn't reflect my style and my passions.

CHAPTER 56

*I*f you have drapes in your home, consider ones that brush the floor. When I moved into my home, the woman who lived here before had exquisite taste. She had replaced all the door handles in the home with gorgeous crystal ones, had painted all the walls in dreamy colors and had hung long luxurious drapes that began near the ceiling and then pooled onto the floor. So glamorous and luxurious! I'd never considered doing this before but I loved the style.

Now, if I ever move I will replicate this. I think it creates an old world luxury.

CHAPTER 57

*M*ake Pinterest your friend. Use it as a vision board. Way to envision your future self.

Instead of cutting out pictures to make a vision board or sitting and imagining a vision of my future life, I get on Pinterest once a week and pin items that reflect the life I want to live.

I have sections for my style, for my future home, for my current home, for a trip I am taking in a few months, for the business I want to have, for the body I want to create and so on.

It's a fun way to do a vision board each week and remind yourself of what you want, who you want to be, and where you want to go.

CHAPTER 58

*C*reate a system to handle your dirty clothes. At the end of the day, all my clothing items have specific places. I have a hanging lingerie bag that zips and goes directly into the washing machine for my lingerie. I hang up items such as my Veronica Beard blazer. I have a regular laundry basket for dirty clothes. I have hooks on the back of my bedroom door for a sweatshirt I wear around the house when I get a chill.

I never throw any item on the floor.

Everything in my wardrobe is handled with care.

CHAPTER 59

*U*se a gua sha.

This is a new part of my morning routine that I briefly mentioned in my section on skin care.

Every morning I squeeze 1-2 drops of olive oil into my palms.

I then pat my palms together and then gently press my palms on my face, neck and decollete. Then I take out my marble gua sha and gently run it along my neck and face in ways that I've studied will help define my face and reduce the puffiness.

There are numerous videos on how to do this and myriad techniques but what I do is run it down my neck. I run it along my jawline. I run it from my marionette lines up to my ear. And I use it to define my cheekbones. I will also occasionally use it under my eyes to reduce any puffiness.

I haven't documented it with photos yet, but I truly believe it does work to tighten and sculpt my face and jaw.

CHAPTER 60

*B*uy small dumbbells or kettlebells and lift weights three
times a week.

If you are a woman, and let's face it, this book is for women,
weight lifting is essential as you grow older. If you've never lifted
weights, start with something small, such as a 3 pound dumbbell and
look up a routine to build muscle.

The earlier you do this the better.

In my humble opinion, lifting weights is the most important thing
we can do (besides walking) to stay in shape and strong.

CHAPTER 61

*H*ost small dinner parties. If it's only a big pot of soup and pillsbury rolls in the oven, do it!

Gathering people together is one of my small pleasures in life.

I learned a long time ago that people don't care if you have a mansion or a studio apartment. People just love getting together. Okay, maybe some awful person would care but why would you want a person like that in your life anyway?

You can also tell people you'll make a huge pot of pasta and ask them to bring wine and bread and dessert. What you serve does not matter. The dishes you serve the food on does not matter. Where you sit does not matter. (Everyone can sit criss-cross style on the floor and be happy.)

Be the one who gathers people. It's a small, simple pleasure in life.

*S*mile at other women.

I make a point to smile at other women when I'm out in public.

I just want to spread support, love and solidarity among women.

Far too many women view each other as competition instead of supporters.

Let's try to change this.

CHAPTER 63

*D*o a financial check up daily.

Every morning I log into my bank accounts and record my balances. Once a month or so I check my larger accounts, such as retirement savings. I know my net worth at any given time. It's worth figuring out your net worth (easy subtract all your liabilities from all your assets and voila!).

I log my expenses and spending each and every day to make sure I am keeping on track with my budget and savings goals.

I also log my income as a self-published author and my royalties from the several publishers who publish the rest of my books.

Staying on top of my finances and loving them in this way has helped me build wealth.

CHAPTER 64

$\mathcal{T}$ake "Me Time" each day.

For me, it's my morning routine and my daily walk. For you, it might be a hot bath or a visit to an exercise class at the gym. Maybe it's lunch with a friend. Whatever small thing you can do that is just for you 100 percent is going to infuse your day with a little extra pleasure.

Carve this time out each day if you can.

It can be something bigger, or something smaller, but make it just for you.

CHAPTER 65

*S*pend time outside each day. No excuses. I live in Minneapolis where temperatures plunge to negative 30 and on those days I may not be outside for long, but I'm outside. Getting light on your face is crucial for your good health.

CHAPTER 66

*D*eclutter your electronics on a monthly basis. Clean up photos, emails, and desktop.

Set a regular time each month to declutter your desktop, your emails, your photos on your phone. Clean this up just like you would clean up your house or declutter your closet.

CHAPTER 67

*T*ip service people well.

Treating those who help us well is just plain human decency but also spreads generosity and love into the world. If you've ever been a service worker, you know how hard some of that work can be. Show your appreciation with your wallet. Take care of others. If you can afford to eat at that restaurant or to take that Uber ride, then you can afford to tip the person providing the service.

CHAPTER 68

*I*f possible, use all natural cleaning products.

This is good for your health and the environment both.

I don't believe you have to buy special products that claim to be all natural.

If you search online you can find ways to kill bacteria and germs with household products such as vinegar and hydrogen peroxide.

Take the time to do a little research and use products that are better for you, mother earth and your wallet.

CHAPTER 69

*S*end thank you cards. In. the. Mail.

I'm astounded by how few people do this nowadays. In fact, I'm astounded by how few people say thank you at all, but that's another subject.

Be classy and send a thank you note or card in the mail for a fun dinner, for a gift, for a favor.

Again, it's about putting love and generosity out into the universe.

CHAPTER 70

*P*rioritize female friendships.

Remember earlier I said smile at other women? Also, make your girlfriends a priority.

I learned this the hard way. I became so wrapped up in raising my kids, my marriage, and building my career that I let friendships go. I regret that deeply and am now trying to rebuild female friendships and I could not value them more. They bring such richness to my life.

CHAPTER 71

*D*evelop a Sunday ritual to prepare for your week.

Mine involves reviewing my journal for the week before and pulling out items I wrote down that I want to remember in the future or that I need to do.

Then I look at my calendar and plan for my week, making note of things to do, appointments and work projects.

When Monday morning rolls around I am organized and energetic and prepared to start my busy week.

CHAPTER 72

*P*lay music in your home.

This is the number one thing I can do to change the atmosphere in my home instantly. I can create a romantic vibe, an energetic house cleaning mood, or even a dance party by simply turning on some music.

Is someone feeling blue? Play happy music.

You can make your home come alive with this simple activity.

CHAPTER 73

*D*iscover what LIGHTS YOU UP. And make time for it on a regular basis.

I keep a list in my head of what lights me up.

Airports. Airplanes. Travel. Exploring new cities. Playing chess. Discovering new restaurants. Walks along the beach. Watching sunsets. Watching sunrises. People watching at sidewalk cafes. Drinking espresso in a coffee shop. Sitting outside in my backyard with a hot cup of coffee and my journal.

So many things. Make your own list and make time to do the items on it.

CHAPTER 74

*C*onsider implementing some affirmations into your routine. Learn about affirmations and consider using them in your day.

You can say them verbally. You can write them down. You can think about them during meditation.

Just research the power of affirmations and consider incorporating them into your own life.

CHAPTER 75

Make your bedroom peaceful and calm. Your bedroom should be for two things: Sleeping and sex. For me, this means no TVs. This means limited electronics. This means soft lights and cozy comfortable fabrics. It means keeping it at the perfect temperature.

Everything is geared toward sleeping or sex.

My bedroom is my inner sanctum, a sacred space.

It is where I go and seek peace.

CHAPTER 76

*L*earn how to be alone.

It is a great gift to be able to enjoy one's own company. I love going to the movies by myself. I love eating at a restaurant by myself. I love traveling by myself.

The list could go on and on.

I love myself. I am confident. And I enjoy being alone with my thoughts.

If you can learn to do this, as well, you will find great peace and freedom.

CHAPTER 77

*R*esearch the water you drink. Sadly, not all water is created equal. Make sure that the water you consume daily is free of harmful ingredients. It's worth spending money to drink water that is better for you or saving up for a filtration system. There is a lot of crap in some water that we definitely don't want in our bodies.

CHAPTER 78

*D*rink lemon water. First thing every morning. I add pink sea salt into mine.

This is something that I truly believe has bolstered my immune system. I make sure to do it every single day. I don't do it with hot water because I want to drink it quickly, but many people put their lemon in hot water and sip that.

CHAPTER 79

*C*onsider picking five meals to eat on a regular basis. Saves money and time.

Lately I've been eating what is called Healthy Keto. On this regiment, my five meals are as follows: An egg omelet with bacon, cream cheese and scallions; a huge salad with tons of vegetables and hard boiled eggs; a steak with asparagus; a piece of broiled salmon with broccoli; a meat and cheese mini platter.

By having these five meals on rotation, I can easily eat healthily and without much thought.

CHAPTER 80

*H*ave impeccable posture. It elevates your entire look. Or bring it down.

It's also good for your health in general. Bad posture not only makes you look dowdy but doesn't allow your insides to function as they should. You don't want to be the older woman walking through the supermarket stooped over do you?

CHAPTER 81

*B*uy organic when it counts.

Learn the Dirty Dozen and make sure you spend your money on buying those items organically.

I used to keep a list of the Dirty Dozen in my phone.

Here are the Dirty Dozen: Strawberries, spinach, kale/collard/mustard greens, peaches, pears, nectarines, apples, grapes, bell and hot peppers, cherries, blueberries, and green beans.

There are also the Clean 15: Avocados, sweet corn, pineapple, onion, papaya, frozen sweet peas, asparagus, honeydew melon, kiwi, cabbage, mushrooms, mangoes, sweet potatoes, watermelon and carrots.

If you forget, a general rule of thumb that usually applies is if something has a thick skin that pesticides are unlikely to penetrate (think avocado or banana) you probably don't need to buy it organically. If it is a food you are eating the skin on, such as an apple or blueberries, organic really counts.

But as you can see from the two lists above this rule doesn't always apply.

CHAPTER 82

*S*eek therapy if you feel helpless, stuck, or just want to improve your life in general.

There is no shame in taking care of your mental health.

Sometimes our problems are just too big to handle alone.

Bring the pleasure back in your life by taking care of and improving your mental health.

CHAPTER 83

*S*tay up on your preventive appointments. Dentist. Annual exam.

I know when I skip my biannual dentist appointment I pay for it the next visit with the hygienist doing a more vigorous cleaning of my teeth.

It's far better to stay up on preventive appointments. Not to mention some of them can save your life.

I've sadly known people who would still be alive today if they had caught something serious earlier during a preventive appointment.

CHAPTER 84

*R*educe. Reuse. Recycle.

Before you throw something away give it a hard look and decide if it can be donated or recycled. We need to protect our resources and use up items before we replace them if possible. That's why it's so important to buy quality over quantity.

CHAPTER 85

Keep an electronic master password list.

I keep a spreadsheet with my passwords on it that I can access on my phone or laptop. This has saved me numerous times.

CHAPTER 86

*D*elegate. It's chic to do so. It's not chic to insist on doing it all. That leads to burnout and possibly a job that could have been done better.

It was really hard for me to learn this lesson.

I like to do it all. I feel competent and independent but I soon realized that true leaders use their time more wisely and focus on what they do best and let others who have expertise take over some tasks.

It's also about prioritizing and spending your time in ways that match your values and bring you the most joy.

For instance, this could mean hiring a housekeeper to come in once a week so you can spend more time with your toddlers.

CHAPTER 87

*C*onsider the one in, one out philosophy.

When you buy a new shirt, get rid of an old one.

If you buy a new book and your bookshelf is packed, get rid of a book you won't miss.

I know this item and philosophy is going to be controversial - "But I need and love my stuff!"

But do you really?

Re-evaluate what you own and what you need.

And yes, sometimes you are going to need all the books on your bookshelves. I get that. But at least consider whether you need something new and if you do, whether you can get rid of something old at the same time.

By thinking this way when you are shopping you are making a pre-emptive strike against clutter, overwhelm and generally having too much stuff.

I'm astonished by the number of people in my city who can't even park their vehicles in the garage during the frigid winters because their garages are full of stuff. So. Much. Stuff.

Avoid this by using the one in, one out philosophy.

CHAPTER 88

aster three recipes.

I think these three recipes are what you need to know inside and out at a bare minimum.

One to whip out when someone arrives at your place unexpectedly. Best if it can feed a group Another if you want to wow someone. And another that is a crowd favorite at potlucks or family gatherings.

Make the first uninvited houseguest recipe something that takes next to zero ingredients or is made from ingredients you always have at home. For instance, I always have pasta, garlic, and parmesan in my house so I can make a giant pot of pasta that tastes amazing in 20 minutes.

If I want to impress something with my limited cooking skills, I have perfected a roast recipe that appeals to everybody I've ever served it to. It's not fancy and I've never met someone who doesn't like a tender cut of meat (well, I'm sure there are vegans who don't but as of right now, none of my friends and family members who eat at my home are vegan so I'm good for now).

The third item is a crowd favorite at potlucks or holidays. For potlucks I bring a meat and cheese board and for holidays I am famous for my garlic mashed potatoes.

CHAPTER 89

*S*tart a book club or trivia team.

I've been in book clubs where nobody has even read the book. And I'm an author. And guess what, I don't care. To me reading and discussing the book is ideal, but ultimately the simple fact that it's an excuse to get together is enough for me.

This past winter, some friends and I started a trivia team where we pick a different bar to go to each week to compete. (Minneapolis has an astounding number of bars that host trivia for some reason.) It has been a ton of fun and a good excuse to get out and see friends on a cold winter night.

*G*et rid of one-trick ponies.

As you go about decluttering your home, ask yourself if you really use and need something that is a one-trick pony. These are often kitchen items that only serve one purpose. Even though I use garlic all the time, I simply use a knife to prepare it instead of a garlic press.

And while I squeeze fresh lemon into a glass of water every single day of my life, I use my hands to do so instead of a lemon juicer.

However, I do occasionally make homemade ice cream for my daughter who has severe allergies and can't eat commercial brands so I do own an ice cream maker, something that someone else might think is a waste of kitchen space.

It's not a one-trick pony if it's something you actually need and use.

CHAPTER 91

*O*rganize a revolving dinner party.

Gather friends or neighbors and organize a revolving dinner party.

One house will provide an aperitif, another can do appetizers, a third neighbor can provide an entree and a fourth can host dessert.

This is loads of fun and a simple way to bring pleasure into your life.

CHAPTER 92

*P*ay attention to your thoughts. Work to eliminate negative thought tracts/patterns.

This is an area where meditation will pay off. The more we learn to become aware of and listen to our thoughts, the greater chance we have of directing our thought patterns to ways that will help us improve as people.

Ridding ourselves of negative self-talk can change our lives.

Be aware of your thoughts and question whether that's what you want running through your mind when you're not really paying attention.

CHAPTER 93

*L*earn tech that can simplify your life. Talking lists to Siri. Alexa.

I often tell Siri to take a note if I'm driving and want to remember something. I might even have her send me an email with something I need to do or know.

I use Alexa to listen to music, to set a timer to meditate, to tell me the weather and to read me the headlines.

I use dictation on my phone to text.

As I mentioned before, my phone alerts me when it is time to start winding down for bedtime. I embrace technology that can simplify my life and I've only touched on the tip of the iceberg of what technology can do for us.

I encourage you to explore this more.

CHAPTER 94

*T*ake care of what you already own. Clean, maintain and resole shoes. Mend minor tears. Fix broken household items that can be fixed. Polish furniture. Fluff pillows. Wax the floors. Keep your oil changed in your vehicles.

You get the idea.

Take care of what you own so it will serve you well and last as long as possible.

CHAPTER 95

$\mathcal{M}$ake sure your house is clean and tidy before you go to bed.

Even if you don't prioritize housework and cleanliness, at least try to straighten up your kitchen and clear your sink of dishes before you go to bed. Do a quick pick up of anything on the floors or surfaces of your house so when you wake in the morning you aren't already feeling behind but can start your day feeling a sense of calm, peace, and organization.

CHAPTER 96

*I*f your life allows it, consider getting a furry friend. I truly believe that one of the most rewarding and rich simple pleasures in my life that absolutely increases the joy in my day is having a dog. In my case, I have two. From the minute I wake in the morning until I tuck into bed with them at night, they bring me enormous pleasure. Their playfulness and unconditional love and devotion is one of life's greatest gifts.

CHAPTER 97

*L*earn how to listen. Hint: it involves shutting your mouth.

Being a good listener is a gift not only for other people but for yourself.

Stopping your thoughts and discarding ideas of what you want to say next and truly listening will expand your world.

In addition, you will gain a reputation as a spectacular conversationalist without barely saying a word as most people interpret someone who is a good listener as a great conversationalist. Go figure.

CHAPTER 98

*D*on't take things personally.

Oh boy if this isn't the secret to life I don't know what is. Kidding. But honestly one of the best possible mentalities to adopt. Realizing that everybody has their own trials and tribulations and that the vast majority of what people say and do only has to do with them and their own lives is absolute freedom. There are a lot of books on how to learn to do this. I'd recommend learning this skill sooner than later.

CHAPTER 99

*B*uy fresh flowers.

Maybe you can't afford to do this every week. Or even every month. I get it. But try to do it every once in a while. Even better, if you have a yard, grow flowers and then bring some inside occasionally.

It's a way, like having plants, to bring nature indoors.

CHAPTER 100

$\mathcal{H}$old an exchange party.

Get your girlfriends together and tell them to bring clothes and accessories and household items that they no longer use.

At the party, people can take turns picking items from the center of the room.

I've been to several of these types of parties and they are lots of fun even if you don't end up taking anything home. (But most people do.)

CHAPTER 101

*L*ive artfully.

Look at your environment as a constant WIP. Constantly curate everything in your life from ridding yourself of toxic friends, to wardrobe and makeup updates.

Your life is a work of art. Live artfully.

Review this book periodically for inspiration.

Add your own items inspired by these.

Remember that you only live once so try to imbue this one precious life with as many simple pleasures as possible.

GRAZIE MILLE for reading my book!
    - Kristi Belle

DISCLAIMER

Be advised that any advice given in this book is simply my own opinion, based on my own experiences. The information included in this book should not be considered legal or financial or medical advice in any way. Please consult with an attorney, doctor or other professional to figure out what is best for you.

This book does not offer any promises or guarantees to your financial security or success. Please consult your own professionals in making decisions.

To the maximum extent permitted by law, this book and Kristi Belle disclaims any and all liability in the event any information, commentary, analysis, opinions, advice and/or recommendations prove to be inaccurate, incomplete or unreliable, or result in any investment or other losses.

Your use of any information in this book is at your own risk.

Printed in Great Britain
by Amazon

23262792R00069